A SPIRITED MOUNTAIN HIKE

A meditative story to massage your body
and relax your mind

BOOKS IN THE NATUREBODY® SERIES

—

Walking in an Ancient Forest

Camping Under the Night Sky

Relaxing by a Waterfall

A Peaceful Winter Ski

Swimming in a Tropical Sea

A Healing Coastal Walk

Relaxing in the High Desert

A Spirited Mountain Hike

The complete
NatureBody® Connection
program is available at

www.aquaterramassage.com

A Spirited MOUNTAIN HIKE

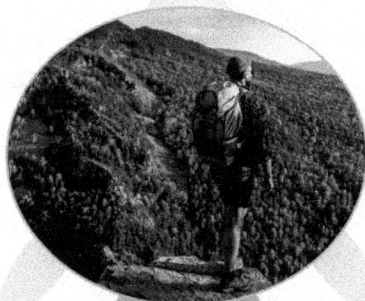

A meditative story to massage your body
and relax your mind

ERIK KRIPPNER *and* FAYE KRIPPNER

Experience the entire NatureBody® Connection at
www.aquaterramassage.com

Dedicated to
those who seek solace
in the mountains.

May you rekindle
your wild and peaceful spirit
in the pages of this story.

Index of Reflections

Contents

How to Use This Book

Humans have lived in balance with our bodies and the earth for 2.6 million years. Our bodies are designed for this planet. It is natural to walk on uneven ground, climb mountains, run long distances, swim, and most of all, to deeply breathe fresh air. Our wild planet heals and strengthens us by making us more flexible and fluid.

Your body is born of this earth. Earth is here to support you. Unfortunately, the stresses of life pull us off balance, and can leave us feeling physically sore and mentally anxious. This creative journey into relaxation is a way to remember your natural balance and create new muscle memories.

As massage therapists, we understand how a relaxed body feels: how it breathes, how it moves, how it is balanced in space. This NatureBody® massage story shares the full spectrum of massage: body, mind and spirit. Our intention is to empower you to find healing within yourself.

Visualization can have powerful effects on your body.[1] In this guided visualization, you will exercise your mind and imagination to deeply relax and bring your body back to center.

If you are injured or your ability to move is limited, then visualization is even more important! Studies have shown that when you imagine moving, the same areas of your brain activate as if you are actually moving those specific muscles.[2] Through visualization, you are virtually exercising your body.

We are intending for you to have a tangible, physical response to the ideas in this book. The power of this story lies in the vividness of your imagination. Read slowly. Pause. Use all of your senses to experience the story. Imagine the changes in humidity. Feel the gentle breeze on your skin. Hear the soothing sound of the wind. Smell the fresh scent of the life around you. Use your vibrant imagination to experience every detail in this story.

Put yourself in the story. Try to experience every sensation in your body. If you feel like moving, do it! Trust your instincts. Imagine what it feels like to move through the story: your muscles warming and stretching... your breathing deepening... your heartbeat slowing as you deeply relax. Let these sensations come to you at the speed of thought. This isn't about concentrating as much as it is about experiencing.

Each time you practice visualizing this story, your experience will become more vibrant. Your body is your wilderness to explore and understand. Your mind is your canvas for new muscle memories.

The Reflections are our personal notes to you. They offer you insight into some of the concepts in the story. Use them to spark your own creative thoughts about connection and healing.

The Notes section is full of wonderful articles and books that we have selected for you. If you feel interested in a topic, we highly recommend you look at the notes to explore the topic further.

The Journal at the end of the book gives you an opportunity to enhance and deepen your meditation. We have asked you a few thought-provoking questions to help you get started. Feel free to write or draw. Journal as creatively as you are inspired. This is your time to dream of the supportive connections between your body and nature.

There is much to discover about your relationship with your body and the beautiful world around you. Find a comfortable place to relax and enjoy. Prepare to be transported to a setting where you can unwind, immersed in nature, and experience the unbridled freedom of the wild!

From Wellness To Oneness,

Erik and Faye
Your Virtual Massage Therapists

FROM WELLNESS TO ONENESS

Wherever you are,

however you feel,

whatever your state of wellness,

know that

healing is at hand.

Your body is always seeking balance

and looking for opportunities to restore.

Through wellness,

may you come to oneness

with your body,

your mind,

your spirit,

and the beautiful Earth that supports us all.

Introduction

We had the privilege to spend two seasons hiking in the Appalachian mountains. The Appalachian Trail runs along this beautiful mountain range, extending 2200 miles from northern Georgia to Maine in the eastern United States. When you dedicate months to being in the wilderness, its life remains in your heart. A part of us will always belong to the Appalachian wilderness, where we lived, wild and free... connected to the seasons, the weather, the forest and its creatures.

The Appalachian Mountain range is one of the oldest in the world. It was created with the formation of Pangaea, when Africa and America collided. The land rippled 30,000 feet into the air, forming colossal mountains. Over time, rain and wind have eroded these mountains into the beautiful, sloping green highlands we see today.

With each step you take in this story, real or imagined, may you find kinship with the land, and your marvelous body.

To experience the entire

NatureBody® Connection

scan this QR code

or go to

www.aquaterramassage.com / naturebodygift / mountainhike

A gift for you, dear reader.

A special reading by the authors awaits you
at the link above.

CHAPTER ONE

Walking through Springtime

LEG MASSAGE AND BALANCE

I am in the heart of the Appalachian wilderness. A narrow trail winds along the valley floor next to a frolicking creek. The honey scent of tulip poplars drifts through the forest.

The world here is colored in the vibrant greens of spring. My eyes absorb the calming green hues and their rejuvenating splendor. It is a beautiful, sunny day: a great day for walking.

Evergreen rhododendron bushes with thick, waxy leaves, cover the hillsides around me. At this low elevation, a few lacy blossoms have emerged. Yet it will be weeks until they are in full bloom. The anticipation of spring fills the air.

The trail is narrow and muddy next to the creek.

*I concentrate on maintaining my balance
over each foot as I step.*

Walking the Line

*"I concentrate on maintaining my balance
over each foot as I step."*

You can keep your balance, even when you are walking on slippery surfaces. Your inner thighs can keep your legs working together so that you are more balanced while moving over the most challenging terrain.

By magnetizing your inner thighs together while you walk, you stabilize each step. Rather than resting into each hip and throwing your balance from side to side, you draw your legs toward your midline, staying centered and lifted throughout your stride. This allows your legs to work together to keep you balanced over your center, which also takes pressure off your hip joints.

Visualize walking on a tightrope. Engage your inner thighs, pulling your legs together strongly. Your weight does not shift from one side to the other. You are directing your energy along the tightrope: firmly balanced over your centerline.

As each foot presses evenly into the ground, your weight pours directly through your arch. This is a more sure and stable way to walk.

Being able to keep your balance over challenging terrain carries over to everything you do. Your strong, coordinated legs can confidently carry you to new places and new activities.

I imagine my legs magnetized together
*   to keep them from slipping.*

My leg muscles firmly spiral around bone.

I am able to walk over slippery surfaces
*   without any feelings of sliding.*

My legs tense and relax fully with each step.

The trail veers away from the stream and begins to climb up the side of the canyon. My breathing increases and my body warms as I head up the trail. The ground under my feet gradually becomes drier and less slippery. My legs relax and my stride lengthens. I am moving fast and sure. My steps are rhythmic, falling in time to my breath and my beating heart.

The creek, now far below, is a silver thread in the basin of the valley. The sound of its frolicking flow has been replaced by a gentle breeze through the trees. The familiar rhododendrons have accompanied me up the hill. Their woody, sinewy branches arch over sections of the path. Long, thin buds of future flowers await their moment to bloom.

My legs are propelling me up the hill.

I place my foot, powerfully pushing
*   with my strong hamstrings and glutes.*

Breathing deeply delivers fresh oxygen to my muscles,
*   warding away fatigue*
*   and keeping them energized.*

My breathing pours oxygen on my muscles
*   like a bellows blowing on a forge.*

Developing Perspiration

"My sweat evaporates, cooling me as my body performs."

Our skin is the largest organ in our body. It is our protective barrier to the outside world. It repels external toxins and shields us from ultraviolet (UV) radiation. Its outer layer cools us by evaporating our perspiration while its inner fatty layer insulates our bodies from sudden changes in temperature.

Perspiring is one of the most vital functions of our skin. Because we sweat, we can more comfortably do the activities that keep us healthy. We can safely go out on a hot day, enjoy a great workout, or spend time in a sauna, because sweating keeps us from overheating.

The cooling effect we get from sweating allows us to perform longer and harder. Anthropologists say that our ability to sweat gave us an advantage in hunting. Sweating allowed us to run long distances so we could exhaust and hunt our prey.[3]

Perspiration, it turns out, is a skill. Our bodies actually develop the ability to sweat more readily as we get in better shape.[4] The more you work out, the less inclined your body is to overheat. You will begin sweating sooner, so that you can work out longer and harder. Don't be afraid to sweat. The more you can do the things you enjoy without overheating, the more likely you are to come to love perspiring!

From the deep shadows of the valley,
    a cool breeze rushes up toward me
    and curls around my legs.

The creek far below is no longer visible. Instead, thick layers of deep green shrubs and trees cover the valley floor.

My legs are warm and glowing
    as circulation flows through them.

My sweat evaporates,
    cooling me as my body performs.

The trail levels out to a long steppe before the final climb to the top of the mountain. The dappled light of the quiet woodland envelops me, hinting of the possibility of sunlit brilliance at the summit.

My breathing relaxes
    and my clear eyes drink in the peaceful surroundings.

The exertion of the climb has calmed
    to the wonder of this new setting.

I am under a canopy of tall and stately trees: tulip poplars with butter-yellow blossoms. Flowers have floated down from the trees in the breeze. I pick up one of the flowers that has fallen into the trail. Its deeply-cupped petals hold a torch of golden stamens.

I inhale its hint of honey.

I exhale happiness.

CHAPTER TWO

High Mountain Meadow

FULL BODY RELAXATION

I am moving at an unhurried, dreamy pace. The sun's golden rays stream through green leaves. A picturesque mountain meadow of fresh green grass opens before me. It is circled by a green-brown woodland with splashes of white dogwood flowers throughout the canopy.

I walk easily across the meadow, my legs still warm from the climb.

I keep my knees bent slightly.

My legs work like springs,
    while my upper body floats observantly above.

My strong muscles support my joints
    as I move fluidly across the meadow.

Breathing Into Tension

*"I patiently breathe into wherever I feel resistance,
allowing inspiration to renew the possibilities in those tissues."*

You can use breath and massage to help release and soften
tense areas in your body.

First, bring your awareness to the tension you are feeling.
Where is the tension? Is it at the surface of your muscles,
or deep in your joints? Is it hot or cold? Dull or sharp?
Can you feel the discomfort radiating to another area of
your body?

Now, begin to breathe, keeping your awareness on that
area of your body. Imagine you are inhaling directly into
the tight tissues, filling them with air. Picture your inhales
gradually expanding the tight area, opening the flow to
these tissues. Imagine your exhales cleansing the area.
Expansion with your inhales. Cleansing with your exhales.

You can enhance this breathing technique by stretching
and moving the tight area of your body while you breathe.
Place a hand on the tight muscle. Visualize the heat of
your hand melting the tissues. Gently massage to soften
them, drawing your deeper strokes toward your heart.

Through breathing and massage, you can communicate
with your body and encourage it to release and relax.

The trail winds through the meadow. I see it disappear into the forest ahead. The meadow is a serene place for renewal. Delicate wildflowers abound among the tender new shoots of grasses.

> *I renew the circulation within me*
> > *by breathing the fresh spring air.*

> *This is the season of awakening.*

In the middle of the meadow, apple trees are just beginning to blossom. I can imagine this beautiful spot later in the season, abundant with fruit. I am happy to be here now, in the cool breezes of early spring.

I sit under an apple tree and remove my shoes. I wiggle my toes, delighting in the freedom from socks and boots. The gentle breeze cools and comforts my hard working feet. Shadows of the tree's leaves dance in the quiet breeze. Sunlight streams down, warming the ground. Birds twitter around me.

> *I lie back.*

> *My low back releases its strength*
> > *and lengthens into a long stretch.*

> *My belly sinks and softens.*

> *I reach my fingertips and toes long*
> > *to stretch my back.*

> *I patiently breathe into wherever I feel resistance,*
> > *allowing inspiration to renew*
> > *the possibilities in those tissues.*

Lengthening Your Neck

"My chin drops down toward my throat
as the back of my neck becomes longer and more graceful."

Many of us deal with tight necks, especially when we are focusing in front of us. We tend to crane our necks forward, off our center of balance. In response, our relatively tiny neck muscles are left to hold up the weight of our heads.[5] This makes our necks tight and sore.

To relax and lengthen your neck muscles, imagine holding an apple under your chin. Let your chin tuck slightly as you lengthen the back of your neck. Lift the crown of your head upward, away from your shoulders.

Breathe, and feel your throat softening in this new position. Pull your shoulders down as your neck lengthens.

With your head balanced over your spine, your neck muscles can release and relax.

As my lungs expand,
   I picture my breath flowing along my lengthening spine.

I imagine gravity
   helping my breath sink down my back.

I am expanding across this earth,
   allowing my body to rest its weight.

My chin drops down toward my throat
   as the back of my neck becomes longer
   and more graceful.

My jaw slackens.

As my muscles release,
   a soft, relaxed warmth flows through my veins.

I lie still, and close my eyes.

I breathe in comfort.

I exhale surrender.

CHAPTER THREE

Ascension

LEG MASSAGE FOR CIRCULATION

On the far side of the meadow, I enter the shade of the forest. Dappled green light streams through the tree canopy. The mountain rises ahead of me. This mountain is part of the Appalachian Mountain range. Time has weathered and worn these ancient mountains to a line of rounded ridges across the earth.

The Appalachian Mountain range was formed millions of years ago when two continents collided. Towering mountains buckled up, taller than the Himalayas. I imagine what this mountain range looked like in its youthful glory: snow-capped, jagged peaks taller than Mt. Everest, soaring tens of thousands of feet over where I now walk. Millions of years of erosion have tempered these lofty peaks. What remains now is the deepest heart of the mountain, the rock most resistant to weathering. I appreciate this ancient earth. The geologic immensity of this place is awe-inspiring.

Unleashing Your Strength

"I ... launch strongly up the trail."

Relaxing your muscles fully can help maximize your strength. If your muscle is tight or sore, some of its fibers are already contracted. It does not have as much strength to give as a muscle that started out fully relaxed.

Think of strength as the combination of tightening and loosening your muscles. We all know that we need to work our muscles in order to become more toned. But we also need to be able to let our muscles go: to relax them fully. The difference between on and off, between fully tightened and fully relaxed, is the amount of power your muscles have available to use.[6]

Ideally, we would have muscles as soft as water balloons. Muscles that are available to contract fully, and then go back to being completely relaxed. They have explosive strength when it comes time to use them, and relaxed flaccidity between contractions.

Massage your muscles. Stretch them. Replenish yourself between workouts. Get the rest, hydration and nutrition that helps your body perform. Encourage your muscles to soften and loosen when you are not using them.

To go from a soft, relaxed, pliable muscle to a strong, fully engaged muscle, is to maximize your strength.

The forest is peaceful, and the soil has grown deep through the millennia. The mountains are thickly covered in abundant and varied life. A rainbow of mushrooms and wildflowers spring up in the soil here. Trees of many species are rooted in the fertile earth. Twisted roots have been exposed on steep parts of the trail, like stairs up the hillside.

My feet conform to the texture of the trail.

I weight them mindfully
and launch powerfully up the path.

As I ascend, I become focused in the moment:
breathing,
walking,
taking in clean air,
allowing my whole body to breathe.

As the heat of my core radiates outward,
perspiration rises and evaporates,
creating a humid aura of cool around me.

I press down strongly on the balls of my feet.
My legs reach out long to receive the trail
while staying grounded and balanced.

The hill ahead is steep. I look to the side to keep my spirits up. Looking forward, I see only the dirt of the rising trail ahead of me. Looking to the side, I see broad valleys and neighboring mountains. I'll know I have reached the peak when I can see light through the trees ahead of me: the promise of the vista to come.

Your Balanced Core

"I use my firm abs to hold my balance back over my feet and offset the lean of my climb."

You can use your core muscles to pull you upright, helping you walk stronger and more freely. When your frame is balanced, your leg muscles can work more fluidly and freely.[7]

Rather than leaning forward to walk, engaging your core helps you balance over your postural center. The muscles around your hips are no longer supporting your posture, but are providing power to propel you forward. By engaging your core, you have more access to your natural strength.

Healthy joints require strong, balanced muscles to move and support them. To lose the muscular support around any joint is to expose that joint to more wear and tear. A balanced posture supports your joints more effectively.[8]

Using hiking poles can help you feel more balanced. They help stabilize your body as you practice new ways of walking. As your balance improves, your poles reassure your new, powerful stride.

It all begins with the core. Your core muscles bring balance to your body and spring to your steps.

I stay in rhythm and keep myself focused,
*   focused on progress,*
*   focused on the moment.*

My legs are long and muscled
*   as I leap up the mountain.*

I lengthen my stride,
*   pushing the trail behind me with each step.*

My strong glutes and thighs
*   power my walk like a steam engine.*

I use my firm abs
*   to hold my balance back over my feet*
*   and offset the lean of my climb.*

I breathe fresh mountain air.

My feet connect with the earth
*   as I lift myself up toward the mountaintop.*

The energy of this walk is peaking,
*   sending circulation racing through my warm tissues.*

My body and breath climb in rhythm.

I begin to see glimpses of light through the trees ahead. The trail levels until I can see light all around me. I have arrived at the summit. A fresh breeze welcomes me, tempering the fire of the climb.

CHAPTER FOUR

Vista

ENERGETIC RECHARGING, STRETCHING THE SPINE

The trees are widely spaced. I feel the warmth of the sun all around me. The trail winds its way across this wide mountaintop. I slow my pace. Waving grasses remind me to be flexible. Weathered rock shows the strength of perseverance.

I catch a glimpse of the incredible view through the trees. I feel higher than this mountain with the sense of accomplishment and gratitude for the infinite beauty around me. The trail leads me out to an open, rocky bluff. Here is my reward for the day's hike. An expansive view spills out in front of me. Forested mountains funnel down to deep green valleys. New spring growth across the land fills the air with warm wisps of living forest incense.

> *I feel freedom in mind and body as I watch*
> *puffy clouds wander across the clear blue sky.*

Shaking off Soreness

*"I check in with my body and shake off
the soreness of the ascent."*

Shaking out your body is a great technique to help relax your muscles. Bounce around and loosely shake your arms and legs. As your muscles begin to relax, you can feel them wobbling back and forth. The more your muscles feel like water balloons, undulating around the bone, the more ready they are for your next activity.

When a task is difficult, we often tighten up, using more muscle than is necessary. This extra muscle tension makes the task at hand even tougher. Shaking is great way to stay relaxed when we are attempting to learn something new, or do something difficult.

Shaking can give you the effect of a deep tissue massage. Feeling your whole muscle move around the bone relaxes muscle fibers deep within the muscle, down to where muscle attaches to bone. Shaking helps remove the extra tension in your muscles.

When your muscles feel soft and floppy, you know they are relaxed and ready to perform.

I remove my boots and stand on the rocky bluff. My legs are amazing. They seem to enjoy working like this. The more I ask of them, the stronger my legs become. I am grateful to have a body that is adaptable and strong.

My body feels wonderful.

I check in with my body
*   and shake off the soreness of the ascent,*
*   shaking my arms and legs,*
*   stretching my neck and spine.*

I bend forward, rolling my spine down
*   one vertebra at a time*
*   until my palms touch the ground in front of me.*

I take a full breath into my spine,
*   and balance my weight evenly*
*   between my feet and hands.*

My head hangs,
*   and I look at the upside-down world behind me.*

Gradually,
*   I shift my weight to my feet*
*   and slowly roll back up to standing.*

I continue stretching,
*   reaching up to the sky*
*   and bending to one side.*

My breath calms
*   and my ribcage opens with my breathing.*

Anchoring to Stretch

*"Keeping my arms raised, I let my shoulders drop
while I stretch my spine upwards into an expansive arch,
looking out to the sky above."*

Building muscle adapts your body to new challenges.
Working out breaks down your muscles. Your body adapts
by strengthening your muscles, creating more fibers than
necessary as it heals them. These extra fibers make your
muscles less flexible. Stretching helps break up those
excess fibers, smoothing and streamlining your muscles.
Stretching muscle is an act of healing.

Small changes in your stretches can make a big difference
to your body. To stretch your spine, gently squeeze your
abdomen and raise your arms up to the sky. Now, with
arms raised, pull your shoulder blades down onto your
back. You are anchoring your arms back into their sockets,
which takes the focus off how high you can lift your hands,
and brings your focus back to stretching your spine. You
are stretching your whole spine from your hips to the top
of your neck. Let the crown of your head rise up while you
anchor your stretch with strong abdominal muscles.
Stretch taller by lifting your abdomen off your hips, and
opening your chest, making more space between your ribs.
These adjustments focus the stretch on your long spine.

With every stretch you do, take time to notice how you
feel. Are your joints anchored in their sockets? Are you
feeling the sense of anchoring to your core while reaching
out of it? Making small adjustments to your stretches can
have a profound impact on how a stretch feels.

I repeat on the other side
to find balance in my body.

Keeping my arms raised,
I let my shoulders drop
while I stretch my spine upwards into an expansive arch,
looking out to the sky above.

My breaths expand my chest wide
and my belly long.

I imagine lengthening my body as I breathe,
adding space between bones.

I close my eyes to feel more deeply.

The reward of stretching is ease of movement
and strength of flow.

With my gentle breath and steady effort,
I attend to feelings of resistance.

As I stretch, I embody
the flowing strength of these mountains.

Here on the mountain, where I have worked my muscles thoroughly and taken the time to relax my mind, my body is easier to hear. I allow myself to be fully awash in the sensations of stretching and breathing. I listen to my body, patiently. My being is cleansed, bathed in the purity of nature.

The Importance of Rest

"I revel in the feeling of being fully present...now."

Resting is an important activity.

Sometimes you know it is time to rest. If you are physically exhausted and it is hard to move, your body may be telling you it needs to take it easy. If it is difficult to concentrate, your mind may be letting you know you need a break. If you are feeling overwhelmed or emotionally triggered by small things, your emotions may be showing you it is time to relax.

It is okay to need rest. Our bodies naturally seek balance. There are times when we are invigorated and energetic, and moments when we need to replenish and restore.

Athletes understand the importance of recovery. They build rest periods into their training. They take breaks between exercises. They alternate between upper and lower body workouts on different days. This gives their muscles the chance to heal between workouts. They actively rest and recover by drinking water and stretching.

Allow yourself time to replenish. Be patient with yourself and your feelings. Give yourself time to heal. Trust that your body will be ready again, and when it is, you will have the energy you need.

I recline back on the rock and open my arms out to the sides. A hawk soars across the sky. With outstretched arms, I feel like I am part of the sky on the open peak of this mountain.

My body widens and lengthens across the ground.
My joints open. My muscles stretch.
Circulation flows freely through me.

I feel my heart beat
and listen to my strong pulse.

I imagine my body opening deeper,
my cells dancing.

I feel as though there are spaces in me
that are letting in the energy of the mountain.

Sunlight and fresh air permeate my being.

As I sit on this peak, looking out to infinity, I think of where I have come from, and where I am going. I have come from a challenging journey of discovery, while ahead of me lie new experiences and adventures. There are more challenging ridges to climb.

I will definitely have a stimulating hike once I leave this serene peak. My muscles will again get warm. I will again breathe hard and sweat and work... fully expressing my body's aliveness here on Earth. But for right now, I am absorbed in this perfect moment, in this idyllic place.

I trust my body will have the strength it needs for the path to come. My spirit springs forth in this season of unbounded energy.

I revel in the feeling of being fully present...*now*.

CHAPTER FIVE

Gratitude

A BLESSING FROM THE MOUNTAIN

T hank you for joining me on this hike. We have climbed from the warm valley to the budding spring heights of the mountaintop. Until we meet again,

May the persistence of mountains
  remind you of your own resilience.

May you breathe
  with the fluid strength of fresh mountain winds.

May the sky of your mind
  remain clear and true.

May the seasons of your life
  sculpt you into a source of strength and serenity for others.

Hike on, Tranquil Wanderer.

Acknowledgments

Thank you to David Krippner, whose strong legs led my early walks and inspired me to hike strong.

I am grateful to the Louisiana, Chitimacha District Boy Scout Troop 231, for introducing me to backpacking and my first hikes on the Appalachian Trail.

To all those whose paths we crossed as we hiked the Appalachian Trail. Your trail names continue to make us smile: Scooby, Sis, River, Chatty Kathy-with-a-K, Sacajawea, Sandstorm, Shine, Animal, Caveman, Spotlight, Bear Boots, Duck Soup, Spot and Starcraft, Bigfoot, Zigzag, Funny Bones, Papillon, Divining Rod, High King, and so many others... You continue to be a colorful light in our stories.

May the sun shine warm upon your face.
May the wind be always at your back.
May the trail rise to meet you.

We, Groove and Bonobo, will always love you.

To Jon Hart, who, among his fascinating lessons on therapeutic massage, boiled it down to "find what is stuck and unstick it." You encouraged us to follow our instincts.

ACKNOWLEDGMENTS

Notes

1. "What is Imagery?" *Johns Hopkins Medicine*, 2003, www.hopkinsmedicine.org/health/wellness-and-prevention/imagery.

2. Lohr, Jim. "Can Visualizing Your Body Doing Something Help You Learn to Do It Better?" *Scientific American*, 1 May 2015, www.scientificamerican.com/article/can-visualizing-your-body-doing-something-help-you-learn-to-do-it-better.

3. Powell, Alvin. "Humans Hot Sweaty Natural Born Runners." *Harvard Gazette*, 19 April 2007, news.harvard.edu/gazette/story/2007/04/humans-hot-sweaty-natural-born-runners.

4. Smith, Paige. "Your Fitness Level May Determine How Much You Sweat." *Huffington Post*, 23 August 2007, www.huffpost.com/entry/sweating-fitness-level_n_5924cdb4e4b0650cc01ff4ff.

5. Fletcher, Jenna. "What Is Forward Head Posture?" *Medical News Today*, 27 February 2021, www.medicalnewstoday.com/articles/forward-head-posture.

6. Charniga, Bud. "The Secret To The Weightlifter's Strength: Speed of Muscle Relaxation." *Sportivny Press*, 30 January 2023, www.sportivnypress.com/2023/the-secret-to-the-weightlifters-strength-speed-of-muscle-relaxation.

7. "How to Walk With Good Posture & Technique." *Wellnessed*, 8 August 2021, wellnessed.com/how-to-walk-with-good-posture.

8. Jonaitis, Jenna. "These 12 Exercises Will Help You Reap the Health Benefits of Good Posture." *Healthline*, 13 April 2020, www.healthline.com/health/fitness-exercise/posture-benefits.

MEDITATION

Journal

This journal gives you a place to reflect on your experience as you read and meditate. With every meditation, your library of personal affirmations can grow. Some thoughts you might want to record, in words or drawings, are:

What were your favorite phrases or ideas in the story?

Did you experience a surge of heat as you imagined climbing from the river valley to the peak of the mountain? What aspects of the mountain did you enjoy the most?

This meditation focused on your hips, legs, and feet. What physical sensations did you notice in your body before, during and after the meditation? How did your breathing change? How did your perspective on walking change?

How have you challenged your body? How did your body respond to the challenges? What adventures do you dream of doing in the future?

"I HAVE COME FROM A CHALLENGING JOURNEY OF DISCOVERY. AHEAD OF ME LIE NEW EXPERIENCES AND ADVENTURES."

MEDITATION

Wherever you are on your path, and whatever is to come, consider for a moment that you have arrived: here and now. Everything you have done and experienced has brought you to this moment. Accept where you are now. Let your breath settle into your belly. Feel it rise and fall with your breathing. Enjoy the "now," feeling connected, tranquil and safe.

~

"AS I ASCEND, I BECOME FOCUSED
ON THE MOMENT: BREATHING,
WALKING, TAKING IN CLEAN AIR,
ALLOWING MY WHOLE BODY TO
BREATHE."

MEDITATION

When it is difficult to shake disruptive thoughts, movement can offer healing. Movement occupies your body and allows your mind to relax, like a moving meditation. The movement can be as simple as the rhythmic cadence of walking, or even the motion of your eyes as you read. Be present with your body and your breath. Let your mind follow your body's cues and enjoy a reprieve from your thoughts.

~

May the

PERSISTENCE

of

MOUNTAINS

remind you

of your own resilience.

"MY BODY WIDENS AND LENGTHENS. MY JOINTS OPEN. MY MUSCLES STRETCH."

MEDITATION

Outdoors, there are no ceilings. There are no walls. There are no expectations. Here, you can stretch long. You can stand tall and proud. You can run freely and rest deeply.

Outdoors, you can laugh loudly. Cry and wail. Holler and snarl and growl. You can truly express your wild, wonderful self.

You belong in nature. You *are* nature. Nurture yourself and embrace your wildness within.

~

"EVERGREEN RHODODENDRON
BUSHES WITH THICK, WAXY
LEAVES, COVER THE HILLSIDES
AROUND ME."

MEDITATION

A rhododendron's leaves are thick and waxy to help protect it from drought. The leaves of this hardy shrub persist through long, dormant winters. In springtime, the rhododendron's blossoms emerge. They are surprisingly lacy and delicate, so different from the thick and hardy leaves.

Like a rhododendron, when you build your own resilience and boundaries to the outside world, you can reveal your gentle, vulnerable qualities.

~

May you

breathe with the

EFFORTLESS

STRENGTH

of

fresh mountain winds.

"I AM ABSORBED IN THIS PERFECT
MOMENT, IN THIS IDYLLIC PLACE."

So often, the perfection of nature delights and amazes us. As we gaze at a flower, or look up at the sky through the soft needles of a pine tree, we are taken by the intricate symmetry, the colors, and the balance of these natural living beings.

Look at your own hands. You are perfectly designed. Can you see the miraculousness of your hands, which can carry heavy loads and yet do the finest and most intricate of tasks?

When we recognize the beauty of nature in our own bodies, we build a compassionate, healing relationship with ourselves and an understanding of our connection to the world around us. We have a natural relationship with nature.

~

"LIGHT AND FRESH AIR
PERMEATE MY BEING."

MEDITATION

Light brings radiance to all that you see. Imagine inhaling fresh air, and accepting warm light deep within your body. Feel it warming and brightening inside you. Allow the light to bring radiance to your tissues. As you breathe, revel in a sense of oneness with the world around you.

~

May the

SKY

of your

MIND

remain clear

and true.

"I AM MOVING AT AN
UNHURRIED, DREAMY PACE."

MEDITATION

Slow down and notice how you are feeling. What sensations are you experiencing? Feel the air on your skin. Become aware of the sensations within your body. Breathe with these evolving feelings.

~

"THE TRAIL FOLLOWS A
CHEERFUL, FROLICKING CREEK
AT THE VALLEY'S FLOOR."

MEDITATION

The movement of the forest is a dance. Trees sway to the wind's music above. Leaves and petals pirouette down to the ground. Water steps and swirls across the stream bed. The contours of the trail lead you in your own choreographed steps along the path. To dance with the Earth is to fully express your aliveness on the planet.

~

May the

SEASONS

of your

LIFE

sculpt you

into a source

of strength and serenity

for others.

"I INHALE A HINT OF HONEY. I
EXHALE HAPPINESS."

MEDITATION

S melling a flower is a joyful, easy way to bring mindfulness into your day. As you bring a flower to your nose, notice its colors and textures. Let the rest of the world fall away as you look at the flower. Now close your eyes and inhale its scent. Breathe in slowly and become awash in this flower's aroma. How do you feel? What sensations do you notice as you breathe the flower's essence?

~

"I PATIENTLY TAKE A BREATH
WHEREVER I FEEL RESISTANCE,
ALLOWING INSPIRATION TO
RENEW THE POSSIBILITIES IN MY
TISSUES."

MEDITATION

As you move, notice how your body feels. What parts of your body are moving well? What parts of your body are feeling restricted?

Focus on an area that feels tight, and imagine breathing into it. Notice how it changes.

You are more powerful than you imagine. No matter what your age or your physical condition, you can relax yourself and find more freedom in your body.

~

BLESSING
FROM THE MOUNTAIN

May the
PERSISTENCE OF MOUNTAINS
Remind you of your own resilience.

May you breathe with the
EFFORTLESS STRENGTH
of fresh mountain winds.

May the
SKY OF YOUR MIND
remain pure and true.

May the
SEASONS OF YOUR LIFE
sculpt you into a source of life and serenity for others.

About the Authors

Born and raised in New Orleans, Erik Krippner grew up with a po'boy in his hand and a song in his heart. As a boy, he spent his summers swimming, hiking, fishing, and sailing. After becoming an Eagle Scout, Erik dreamed of answering the call to "Go West, young man." He earned a Bachelor of Science degree in Forestry from Louisiana State University. Following his passion for adventure, Erik found his way to the mountains of the Pacific Northwest, his home to this day. After working in the forests of Oregon, Washington, Idaho, Alaska, Georgia, and Louisiana, Erik decided to focus his love of natural sciences on the study of human body through massage therapy.

Faye grew up in Oregon surrounded by family and old growth coastal forests. She spent many childhood weekends cross-country skiing, hunting for mushrooms, exploring coastal tide pools, and searching for crawdads in the Siuslaw River. Her love of books deepened when she became the editor of her high school and college's literary journals. Upon earning her Bachelor of Arts degree in Mathematics with honors from the Robert D. Clark Honors College at the University of Oregon, Faye became a technical writer and web developer. The whisper of a deeper purpose ignited her to study massage, where she met Erik.

Erik and Faye became friends in massage school at the East West College of the Healing Arts, in Portland, Oregon. In 2003, they founded Aqua Terra Massage, a therapeutic massage studio for friends and couples. Since then, they have practiced therapeutic massage together, side by side. They have spent years immersed in the study of massage, serving thousands of clients.

Faye and Erik have spent years exploring and writing about our beautiful world. They have sailed the blue waters of Fiji's Koro Sea, kayaked New Zealand's Marlborough Sound, and stargazed among the giraffes and elephants in Botswana. They have hiked the Appalachian Trail and paddled the tidally-influenced Columbia River in the Pacific Northwest. They have seen orca whales swim right under their kayaks, locked eyes with wild lions, and played hide-and-seek with an octopus. They have hiked thousands of miles together, kayaked and sailed hundreds, and spent countless evenings camping under the stars.

With a commitment to bringing more love and kindness
to this beautiful world, we offer this book to you.

www.aquaterramassage.com